Another Little #1 Secret that Diet Gurus Don't Want You to Know

(Diets Don't Work So Stop Hitting Your Head Against the Wall!)

Table of Contents

Dedication

This book is dedicated to my husband, the "Food Nazi". Without your obsession with what's in our food, I would've never been able to write this book. See, I WAS paying attention after all!

Disclaimer

Standard disclaimer applies: I'm no expert, I don't have a degree in nutrition, I don't take responsibility for your health and neither should anyone else except, YOU! So, that said, let's go!

Introduction

So, you've mastered the art of moving and are once again svelte and thin right? No? What happened? I'll tell you what happened. Life! That's the way life goes, and trends and gimmicks and all of the other little things that we fall for every day.

I'm here to help you wade through all of the muck and mire (is that a real word?) and help you find your happy weight. Not your happy plate, although we could go over that too.

My hubby and I have gained and lost so much weight that we could've had a whole other person living with us right now. We could call him Tub O' Goo. That's not to say we've mastered anything yet, but it's the journey that we're on that we felt we would like to share with you now.

This book will help you change, not only the way you eat, but how you think about food. It will help you determine what is **REAL FOOD!**

Let me say this before we ever get started, **I LOVE FOOD!** I love to cook for my family and friends and I especially love to cook extra special foods for holidays. So, we are going on this journey together once again. Oh, and let me add this, if it tastes like cardboard, **I WON'T EAT IT!** Okay, so let's get started.

Use Your Brain Before You Eat

(Engage your brain before engaging your mouth)

"Whatever you hold in your mind on a consistent basis is Exactly what you will experience in your LIFE" –
Anthony Robbins

This little book is very similar to the previous "Secret" book in that the hardest thing to change is your mind about how and what you eat. I've read and watched and purchased tens of things (I didn't want to exaggerate and say hundreds) that are supposed to be the best and latest thing to losing weight. I've bought pills and vitamins and supplements. I've made cabbage soup, and drinks made from Swiss chard and hazelnuts. I've choked down my share of cardboard microwavable meals. Sure, maybe I lost a few lbs here and there, but it was probably just water weight from the adverse effects of my poor stomach having to unload the barrage of weird things I was putting into it. Believe me when I say, I've pretty much tried it all.

So let's put away all the stuff we've done and learned before and now we can start fresh. As I said before, I love food. I was a foodie before there was a term foodie. I can still conjure up the smell and taste of my mom's roast beef and mashed potatoes with good brown gravy. Or how about fried chicken? See how easy it is to divert down that old rabbit hole? I was raised on the basic food groups. Meat, potatoes, salad and homemade bread, oh and don't forget the dessert. I recall one time when I was probably a teenager and I really didn't want to have dessert.

My mom insisted saying, "You need to do your part and eat this up." We had a good laugh over this, and still do once in awhile, but I really think things like that are at the core of what is wrong with my thinking about food.

Now I live with my husband, whom I lovingly call the "Food Nazi". He just laughs and continues to insist I read labels at the store and makes me watch food documentaries and can generally be a pain in the neck. But, he's right. Please don't tell him I said that. I will never hear the end of it.

Changing your mind about food is like any other habit you have, YOU HAVE TO WANT TO CHANGE!

A few years ago the hubster and I started a weight loss challenge with each other and another gal that worked for us at the time. Right before we decided to do this I had seen a video of myself in a concert. WOW! That was enough to motivate me!

We had a great time during this contest (I won by the way!) and lost 40+ pounds in the process. We kept it off for over a year, then we had some financial difficulties and each had to get real jobs. That completely messed up our diet and exercise routine. So the weight started packing on again. I will explain how that happens in a later chapter.

Well, a few weeks ago, I went with my daughter-in-law to take my granddaughter to an interactive fountain. I volunteered to chase baby girl and she took video with my phone. I watched in horror afterwards as images of myself appeared on the screen. That was another of those life changing moments when you want to crawl in a cave and never come out (until the next meal is served.)

Here is the really scary part. I've been moving and walking and doing all of the things I told you to do, but I looked bigger than I had ever seen myself. We had even been watching our diet, drinking homemade juices, eating veggies and whole grains.

That's when a HUGE (pardon the pun) light bulb went off in my head. Something else is making me fat. Seriously, we don't over eat (except on occasion) and I'm still gaining weight.

Okay, two things happened. First I got on the computer and started searching about thyroid disease. I almost decided it must be my thyroid, or maybe menopause. Then I realized my hubby hasn't lost an ounce either. So, how could we both be gaining without overeating? Well, duh! It's our food. We both felt bloated much of the time and neither of us had much energy or oomph for the things we usually love to do, like garden, killing bugs or shooting wasps with water. Even making fun of the tourists that ride by on their bikes has lost its appeal.

The second thing I realized is this; I can't picture myself looking slender and healthy. What I had been doing was to only do a check-up from the neck up. I was pretending that I was alright, when in fact I wasn't even feeling alright, much less looking alright. I know we have to accept our bodies and blaa, blaa, blaa. I'm really okay with that, but when you're not feeling healthy, you **don't** have to accept that.

So, after doing my research, I sat myself down and had a heart to heart talk. I said, "Self, no one is going to do this, but you. You can't depend on the Food Nazi to always make choices for you, so now is the time to change your mind."

Nothing, nothing, nothing can change unless you change your mind first. Let me say that again. NOTHING is going to CHANGE unless YOU

CHANGE your MIND! If you're happy with your weight and body, then more power to you. But I really want to be able to fit into the other 95% of my clothes hanging in my closet.

I blamed "Global Warming", coming in and shrinking all of my clothes when I wasn't looking. I know, lame.

But Mostly I want to feel good. I want to be able to chase grandkids around the yard or get up from playing on the floor without feeling like my knees are going to give out any moment.

So, how do we do this? First you have to want to change, like I said before. Then you have to picture yourself already changed. Okay, so here's where we get weird. Your mind is the most powerful tool you have. I know that anything you tell yourself will come true if you believe it.

One of my favorite quotes is from Henry Ford that says, *"Whether you think you can, or whether you think you can't, you're right."*

You have to believe yourself already slender and healthy. A few years ago I read in a magazine that if you're trying to lose weight you should find a picture of the body you want and put your head on the picture and post it somewhere that you will see every day. I probably just dismissed that as rubbish. I wish now that I had paid attention. I would've been that much closer to getting this whole thing right. This time I picked out a smokin' hot body and I can't WAIT to see me in it!

The next thing you should do is to go shopping for an outfit that you want to fit into. Or if you're not sure about what size you'll end up, just cut a picture out of a catalog, or magazine.

Picture yourself already in the outfit. Feel the snugness of the jeans, listen to the sound of the zipper as it easily moves, smell the new denim, see yourself in the mirror (front and back) and how great these new jeans fit. Taste the victory on your tongue.

Or maybe it's a different kind of goal, like hiking the Grand Canyon. I suggest you put a picture of someone on the trail that you will someday be on. You need to picture yourself walking down that trail. Feeling the wind on your face, smelling the mules sweat as they pass by you, taste the cool water as you get a drink from your canteen, hear the eagles cry down the canyon, and take in the beautiful view as you move further and further towards your goal. I know it sounds a little hokey, but it really works.

Another step to using your brain is to tell your body that you are already slender or healthy. This doesn't mean you are in denial. What it means is that you believe **you will** meet your goal. You have to feel and want to **BE** slender and healthy. If you continue to accept poor health and being overweight, your body will go along with what you are telling it to do. This is the one place where you are master and commander of the universe. YOUR universe is your body. Leaving everything to chance is like letting every enemy come into your borders and running all willy nilly over you.

Trust me, this is going to take some practice, if you're like most of us, we've been on auto-pilot for most of our lives and now you have to take back the controls.

A History of What We Call Food And Why We're Fat Now

"You're programmed to put on fat whenever food is available." Dr. Christine Northrup

Now that you've made up your mind to be healthy and not overweight, you've got to make sure you know **HOW** to eat, and **WHY** to eat this and not that. As I said earlier, I've tried almost every fad diet and gimmick that's out there. I've watched infomercials and purchased pills and potions till I could start my own diet store. Instead, I'm going to give you all of my research and knowledge in a few easy steps.

First of all you need to know that none of your less than stellar finishes were your fault. It has nothing to do with lack of willpower, or lack of desire, or even how much you have eaten! It has to do with the kinds of food we were told to eat and when to eat them.

I have come to the conclusion that not only was I eating the "wrong" healthy foods, but I wasn't eating enough food, period.

Your body is made up basically of just four elements: oxygen, nitrogen, carbon and hydrogen, most of these in the form of water. Sounds pretty simple right? Well, it can be, but what we have done is complicate everything by putting "fake" foods into our systems. Our bodies are bombarded daily with chemicals and additives and so-called foods that it has to deal with, and it may just store them up as fats to use later.

Back in the day, our grandparents, and some of our parents grew their own food down on the farm. They had gardens, chickens, cows for milk and meat, pigs and every fresh food you could imagine. Somewhere along the way, the family farms were plowed under to make new suburban homes and shopping malls. Fewer and fewer farms were expected to feed more and more people. In order to feed the demand, farms became a part of a huge conglomerate, agri-business, instead of fulfilling small individual needs, they were a part of a large farming machine. I'm sure our grandparents and their parents wouldn't recognize a farm as it is today.

Okay, back to the wrong "healthy" foods. Those big, bad corporations came up with an ingenious idea. They would modify the seed, so that the grain would be resistant to pests, or change what color the corn comes out so it's more attractive. They also changed the outcome of what used to be a veggie – it is now "food-like," but not real, natural food in its whole original state.

This is called genetic modification or genetic engineering. By changing the outcome of a fruit or vegetable, they can receive a patent. If they have a patent on the seed they have the rights to who uses it.

Farmers used to harvest their crops and then save back seed (if possible) for the next year's crop. Now that the big corporations have these patents, even if the pollen from this seed mixes with another, they will own that new mixture as well. Thus forcing many farmers to buy seed from big corporation seed companies and that in itself has lead to part of the dilemma we have today.

Genetically modified organisms or GMO's are everywhere! If you think you are eating healthy by eating whole grain wheat, soy or corn, think again. Anytime you mess with the genetics of a plant, it becomes man made. If it's not organic to our bodies, our body may not know what to do with it.

In the United States and Canada, food producers are not required to put GMO labels on packaging. Most European countries now require these labels. It's not only wheat that's been changed, its soy beans too, but the most blatant of changes has happened with corn. Lately, the corn supporters have been bombarding us with commercials letting us know that corn syrup in things is okay. Wrong again! Corn as corn is ok, but once you change its form, into corn syrup, it's no longer a real food. It becomes a concentrated sugar.

Let's take, for example, the adding of high fructose corn syrup in our food. This is just another fancy word for sugar or sweetener. Once the sugar is ingested it turns to fat. This doesn't happen immediately, what happens is that once you take in this sugar, it sends your blood sugar levels up. When your blood sugar levels go up, the pancreas produces insulin. Insulin is the hormone that delivers glucose (or sugars) to your cells for energy. When you have a spike in your blood sugar, the pancreas sends insulin in to bring levels back down to a normal range. This can cause a blood sugar crash. If you've ever had a pop and you feel the high. Then about 10 minutes later, you feel either dead tired or you are starving. This is your body trying to regulate your blood sugars. This can go into a roller coaster effect if your blood sugar doesn't get regulated right away. It may eventually be stored as fat if it can't process the sugar for fuel. This is what's called type 2 Diabetes.

So, you say, "I don't eat sugar, at all." Well, I think you'd be surprised at how much sugar you actually eat without ever spooning any on your cereal. Take for instance your cereal. Take a look at the box and check out how many sugars there are on it. The "whole grain" cereal in itself turns to sugars in your body once you've ingested it. Bread, cereal, breakfast bars, juice, most everything you consume for breakfast turns right to sugar, and too much sugar is stored as fat. Hmm, now I have your attention, don't I?

A better option might be some organic oatmeal, spelt bread toast or even the ancient grain quinoa with honey.

Don't forget the "low fat, or "no fat" options. Yes, they may be lower in fat, but they've loaded them up with more sugars, which turns to fat! See what I mean?

So, you say, I use artificial sweeteners, I'm good. Sorry, not so fast. Just wait till I tell you how artificial sweeteners are making you fat! Diet soda? Forget about it. I will explain that in a later chapter.

When they isolate certain parts of a plant, it can become toxic or even deadly. Take for example the coca plant. If it's used as a whole for, let's say coca plant tea, it's perfectly okay. But if you separate and isolate certain chemicals in that plant, you get the highly addictive drug, cocaine. When they isolate and separate corn syrup from corn, you get a food-like substance that is used in most "prepackaged, processed, prepared foods". Just look at everything from cereal, to fruit juice or crackers, or even pizza sauce…it's in there. It's almost exclusively in soda pop. They are now making some pops that are called "Throw back" in these they use "real" sugar; which is processed white sugar, NOT real sugar.

Why you ask? I'm glad you asked. Well, because it enhances the flavor. Really? I'm pretty sure it only makes it taste sweeter. Why would we want things to taste sweeter? Hmm, let's see…. to feed our addiction. Not only are we addicted to sweet things, but Americans are addicted to cheap food. The food industry has found a way to give us just that. If you've ever tried to buy "healthy food" on a budget, you know exactly what I'm talking about. You can get boxed mac and cheese for less than a dollar a package, but oranges and apples are a dollar a piece.

The United States Government is complicit in this. In the 1930's the government actually paid farmers to let their fields lay fallow, this was done to limit the amount of corn grown to keep prices high. Then in the 1970's they did away with that and changed it in order for farmers to expand and grow as much as they could. What this did was paved the way for corporations to take over the farming industry. The mom and pop farmers were squeezed out in order for the big boys to take over.

Farmers are still paid a government subsidy to grow a commodity crop. Without that, the farmers would lose money growing these crops. Now corn is grown for more than the vegetable corn. It's grown for the food substitutes and addictive properties of high fructose corn syrup. The government pays the farmers the difference between a market price and the deflated price. That way they can drive the cost of food in whatever direction they want to.

Even the US Department of Agriculture admits in one of their studies, "The average American consumes more than 150 pounds of sugar and sweeteners each year."

A quote from Alejandor Junger, the author of "Clean" says, *We are not eating food anymore, we are eating food-like products and they are adorned, made to look better and smell better, so that people are attracted to them."*

If you stop and think about that, it's really kind of sad, people have to be "tricked" into liking a food?

There's more to it than that, the food is made with certain ingredients to keep us coming back for more. Just like cigarettes, food is now made to create addictions, so that the food industry will profit and we will become slaves to it.

Once upon a time we had a built-in food-o-meter. Our bodies had great survival instincts and we knew how and what to eat and when. All through history the big challenge was to find enough calories to survive the coming famine, or winter or next big time we would have a scarcity. We would seek out calories and fats to sustain us through those times. It's kind of like a bear, who knows instinctively to fatten up in the fall for the big sleep. Human bodies were put through the same kind of stresses. After the time of stress was over, their bodies sought to replace those things that were lost during that time.

Now our bodies still have that built-in instinct to protect us from these stresses of famine. So when we taste something sweet or fatty, our brain tells us, " I want more." Because for our ancestors, this meant survival to prepare for the lean times.

The only difference is that your body doesn't know if this was a self-imposed stress or not. So, just in case, it tells you to put on an extra 10-20 pounds to get ready for the next famine. This is the exact reason that after dieting, most people put on extra weight after they stop the fast.

So, now what? We no longer have famine, we have a constant supply of food, but we have no way to deal with it all.

The best way to explain how to conquer this is to eliminate certain foods and to add others. In order for this to work well, you must do this in a careful, calculated way, in order for your body to assimilate to it gradually. That way your body isn't stressed and thinking it needs to over compensate for the lack of food. Enough of history, let's move on to a "new you".

Living With A Food Nazi

"Nothing tastes as good as being skinny feels."-
Kate Moss

"Pizza tastes as good as being skinny feels."-
Lauren Leto

I realize that not all of you are as fortunate as I am to live with a food Nazi. Unfortunately you will have to be your own watchdog so to speak.

My husband would bring up things about what we were eating at the dinner table, and in some instances, refuse to eat certain foods. This was particularly upsetting to my mom who loves to cook for us. I finally got him to stop, and either eat what she served, or politely pass it on.

The hardest part for me was shopping on a budget. You have to watch your pennies, as well as read every label in the store. I finally decided to stop fighting him and check these things out for myself. After reading more than a few articles, and books and watching some documentaries, I made up my own mind.

It didn't really hit me until, as I said earlier, I was fat and nothing I did was changing that. Then, and only then, was I really interested in what I was eating.

All joking aside, I am really thankful that my husband has taken the time and effort to continue to get to the truth about nutrition and food.

He has been saying he's a vegetarian since I met him nearly 20 years ago. Well, he would still eat pepperoni pizza and hot dogs. How those two things factor in to a vegetarian diet, I'm not exactly sure. But never the less, he's tried to stay away from meat.

Recently, I have been able to present some of the cold hard facts about processed meats to him, so our pepperoni and hot dog diet has all but diminished. In fact, since he's gotten me started, we now share information and new documentaries that might be useful in our quest.

Yes, I blame him for this, but I think he may have been saving our lives.

It's Not What You're Eating—It's What's Eating YOU!!!!

"Let food be thy medicine and medicine be thy food"
Hippocrates

When you become a person of a certain age, your health starts to become a factor as well as the worry of being overweight. In fact, the two sometimes go hand in hand.

Sugar

I was never one of those people who freaks out about chemicals and cancer, but when I found out that every person has cancer cells in their body, I sat up and paid attention. Then, I found out cancer LOVES sugar. This is not to say, sugar causes cancer directly. But, indirectly sugar adds to weight gain and if you are overweight you are more likely to get diseases like cancer, heart disease, and diabetes. But, if you <u>do</u> have cancer, don't eat sugar!

A study at the University of London used a new cancer detection method with an MRI. The MRI is used to detect glucose in the body, these cancer tumors light up like Christmas trees, because they contain high amounts of glucose, or sugar.

My brother was diagnosed with cancer a few years back and HE has become a quiet food Nazi. No, make that, nutrition advocate. He is an advocate for his own health. He doesn't eat sugar, or sugar substitutes and after his initial detox from sugar, even fruit is too sweet for him.

There are numerous studies that are now confirming the fact that many more diseases are directly connected to sugar consumption.

A study by Dr. Robert H. Lustig, M.D., a Professor of Pediatrics in the Division of Endocrinology at the University of California, San Francisco, states that the majority of chronic illnesses that we have today are in direct response to our sugar intake.

Not only is sugar bad for you, but those wonderful little sugar substitutes are just as bad, or even worse.

Aspartame is now found in most "diet" foods. Aspartame contains chemicals that actually kill brain cells. When you combine this with caffeine, it's a deadly match. Diet soda has become a staple for many people trying to lose weight. After consuming the drink, you feel a "high". This is the caffeine hitting your brain cells right before they die. Kind of like the finale in a fireworks show, going out with a bang.

"So what?" you say, "Brain cells die all of the time."

You're right, of course, but once again it can make you fat. Aspartame creates cravings for carbohydrates. Hmm, like chips, cookies and fries. So, all those calories you saved by drinking a "diet" drink are not only canceled out, they are completely obliterated by the consumption of more carbs than your body needs in a day.

Drinking diet soda can also lead to having cognitive problems, headaches, visual problems. Here's a partial list of what aspartame can do to you. Nausea, vertigo, insomnia, blindness, memory loss, depression, joint pain, hearing loss and can even lead to different kinds of cancer.

Commercial pilots are discouraged to drink this because of these well known factors. Makes you think huh?

Monosodium glutamate, or MSG is used in processed foods to add flavor. It's not only used in most Chinese foods, but in more than 75% of all processed foods.

MSG has been found to give migraine sufferers headaches, so it's to be avoided if possible. I found this out at least twenty years ago. So, being a person who gets migraines, I started being very careful about this additive. Recently I found out that MSG is now on labels under some fifty plus other aliases, so that throws that right out the door.

Another use for MSG has been to determine how food makes lab rats fat. In fact, if you look up "fat rats" on the internet, it almost exclusively has to do with how much MSG they were fed in order to get the results they were looking for.

Propylene glycol is a chemical used by the food industry to make "pretend blueberries" among other things. No big deal right? Not so fast.

Propylene glycol is used to winterize RV's, you know, **anti-freeze.**

Fats, can be bad. Not just any fats, but partially-hydrogenated fats, the fats that are in oils like soybean oil, and especially canola oil. Canola oil, over a long period of time can cause numerous problems. Fake butter, margarine and shortening are three fats that are commonly found in most American kitchens.

Margarine is made by using chemically extracted vegetable oil. The oil is extracted at high temperatures which damages this already poor quality product even further. In order to make margarine, the oil has to be hardened. This is done by bubbling hydrogen through the vegetable oil. The hydrogen then saturates the bonds of the oil and it becomes hard. This is called a "saturated fat."

For quite awhile now, researches have known that saturated fats can be harmful to the body. They found that these fats can clog your arteries and also activate enzymes that may develop insulin resistance. Back to that again? Yes, this can lead to type 2 diabetes.

Processed foods **CAN** and possibly **WILL** kill you. Or at the very least make you fat....

Food Addictions and

Food Smut on Social Media

"The trouble with eating Italian is that 5 or 6 days later, you're hungry again."- George Miller

Americans love to love things. We love movies, we love cars, we love certain foods, and most of all we love convenience. Oh, and I almost forgot, cheap things, mostly cheap food. These loves, soon turn to obsessions and addictions.

I have to admit, I love to look at food and dream about making those luscious brownies, or drool over that cheesy, potato casserole. I shared these recipes on social networks, not to steer anyone away from eating right, but in hopes that I could somehow re-work the ingredients to make it healthy. In doing this, I found out I was actually not helping others who, like me, have food addictions. It's like taking an alcoholic to a bar and asking them to sit while you have a drink. Some people can just look and walk away, some can't resist. So, for that, I apologize. I will no longer share food smut on social media. Well, maybe once in awhile.

Diet Soda

As I stated in the previous chapter, diet soda can make you not only fat, but can kill you as well. I've known people who don't eat food, they just drink diet soda and eat chips or candy all day. They are consuming "empty calories." A woman I used to work with, was tall and lean and looked like she was healthy. But, if you looked closer you could see how tired and haggard she really looked. She was starving her body of nutrients, just barely surviving on one real meal a day. She had a heart attack at the age of 48 and afterwards she told me that she would never do that to herself again. She's gained weight, stopped smoking and looks and feels much better.

Her addiction to diet soda, tricked her into thinking she didn't need anything else.

Fast Food

Okay, so I have been as guilty as the next person about this. I used to LOVE tacos and hamburgers on the go. I still grab one every once in awhile to remind myself why I don't eat this stuff anymore. It literally makes me sick.

A few years ago we learned that the American Fast Food industry was adding low cost filler into the hamburgers available at most fast food restaurants. This is called "Pink Slime."

What they do in order to make this, is shave the bones, take the rejected fats, parts and scraps from the meat packaging process and make it into a low cost meat additive. This product was sold to dog food makers until recently when our addictions demanded low cost food. How do you think they can keep the dollar menu alive?

Not only are there scraps of meat in this stuff, they add ammonia in order to kill the bacteria that this stuff is full of. And many times ammonia doesn't kill the bacteria.

I just found out that the pink slime is not limited to fast food, but is found in many ground beef packages available in your local grocery store as well.

A better bet would be to buy from a local rancher, organic if possible, and grass fed. I watched another documentary that showed how cows are now fed, in order to make the meat cheap…aka affordable. Not only are cattle fed a constant diet of corn, cheap corn, but in one instance a farmer bought old Halloween candy and fed it to his animals. Pure sugar, no nutritive value. No wonder they have to pump antibiotics into the poor cows.

I have a friend who contracted a rare infection and when she went to her doctor for help, he prescribed a typical antibiotic. This did not help, in fact she got worse. They gave her a stronger dose, still nothing. After a very scary few months and a close call of dying, they finally gave her a medicine that cost close to $5,000. This woman takes care of kids for a living, so this was a big burden for her.

After this was all over with, her doctor asked her if she had taken lots of antibiotics as a child. Her answer was, "Never!" So where did the resistance come from? The only answer was from what she had consumed in her life. Not only are the bugs getting bigger and more resistant to drugs, but our own bodies are no longer able to take antibiotics due to eating them in our food supply every day. Makes you stop and think a bit.

Salt- Sodium

Salt is a necessary element for our body, but the recommended amount, (less than 6g) per day is just a fraction of what most people ingest every day.

Salt is used by the body for digestion, helps to regulate fluids in the body and help to maintain a level PH balance. However, we consume way, way too much. The problem goes right back to the processed foods, they add sodium, salt and monosodium glutamate right from the start. Not to mention fast foods or pizza. Next time you eat a meal that is prepared before you get it, pay attention to your hands and feet. My hands nearly always swell after I eat pizza or fast food, especially French fries.

These are obvious side effects of too much salt, but some of the underlying effects can be hypertension (high blood pressure), osteoporosis, and even stomach cancer.

Stop Thinking in Terms of Die-t

"I've been on a diet for two weeks and all I've lost is two weeks."-

Totie Fields

Okay, so now what? What do we do with all this information? What CAN I eat?

Well, this goes back to your mind re-set. You have to think in terms of "I **can** eat that, but I choose to eat something better."

Instead of restricting bad, just add more good. In my first book, I joked about cleaning out the fridge and cupboards. This is a very helpful tip. I am a person who can go all day eating right, then about 5 o'clock, I start to graze. I will eat anything not tied down. I can make even the healthiest foods into something not so good. If I find raisins and nuts, I will add old marshmallos and chocolate chips to them, just to satisfy my cravings.

The problem is, this doesn't satisfy me, it only adds to my craving. If I have a sweet, then I want a salty and it goes on and on.

What's really happening here is that my body is trying to find the nutrients it needs. I probably need magnesium, thus the chocolate. Your body will continue to send you signals until you get it right. In the meantime, you've plowed through tons of unwanted calories and empty food-like items.

That's why when you wolf down a burger and fries, you still want more. You haven't satisfied your body's nutritional cravings.

Once you get rid of most of your "bad foods", you can start adding good ones in. That way if you have a problem with chips or candy and cookies, they are no longer there to tempt you.

Now, that said, don't beat yourself up if occasionally you do have a treat. I hate going to a BBQ or dinner and thinking I can't eat anything there. Once in a while it won't hurt you. But if you are an addict, you must know what your triggers are. If you can't pass up a plate of brownies, and this is going to send you into a sugar bender, then stop yourself. Get to know your own body and what it can handle. I still think it's better to allow yourself a treat once in a while, or you'll drive yourself crazy thinking about it. It might lead you to go off the wagon.

After getting your kitchen ready, I would recommend a detox from sugar, and all the preservatives that have been invading your body for a while now. The easiest way I know is to do a juice cleanse. If you have access to a juicer, fresh juice is best. If not, I would highly recommend buying one as soon as you can. You can pick one up at the store for under $100. These juicers aren't the high quality you might need in the future, but for now this will work.

If you've never done a cleanse, you might not feel so good right at first. You could have headaches (withdrawl from sugar and or caffeine) and you might feel like you're starving to death. You aren't and you will get through this and trust me, after a few days you will feel so much better. I did a partial cleanse over a year ago, (I had some protein like nuts once a day.) Most experts recommend doing this every 90 days or so. I would suggest trying a three day cleanse first. If you do ok, you could continue for another few days. Probably no more than that though.

Once you are through it, you will start to feel much better. You will notice you can think clearly and you actually feel satisfied when you eat or drink. You will also find that you crave the "right" foods, like salads and raw foods.

A few years ago when my husband and I were trying to find a business to add to our income, we happened upon a supplement company that extols the benefits of juicing. They believed it was too hard to get all the vitamins and nutrients from juice alone, so they sold a supplement to help with that. We were just getting started in this arena, so when we were invited to a "BBQ", I wondered how this was going to work. The majority of the folks were vegans, so it was raw food. I thought I was going to starve. Of course I didn't and it's pretty close to the way we eat now.

One woman shared that since they had started eating this way, her teenage son was now craving things like salad and carrot sticks instead of burgers and fries. I dismissed that as a sales gimmick and went home and ate some "real" food.

Now, five years later, I know this can be true. I'm not saying everyone has to be a vegan, or eat all raw foods. No, you have to determine what is right for you and your body. If you still want meat, try for organic and "free range". Just become aware of what you put in your mouth and know that we can no longer mindlessly wander the aisles of the grocery store and trust that everything in there is okay to eat. You have to take charge of your own health, whatever that means.

If you do adopt the vegetarian or vegan lifestyle, you might be pleasantly surprised at some of the perks. You don't have to cook very often! You can drink a nice juice for dinner and add some protein like cheese or nuts.

One of the benefits of drinking juice and eating more raw foods is that you might actually feel "satisfied." You might not always feel full, but more times than not, you will feel refreshed and satisfied. Once you get your body in balance you will actually be able to "feel hungry."

Some people have never felt what it really feels like to be hungry for food, not just the urgency of filling up with calories and salt to stop your cravings.

Another thing I suggest is to make two lists. These two lists are of all the "good foods" and "bad foods" you like. For instance, I love watermelon, but then again I love Peanut Butter milkshakes. After completing both lists, go over them and see what you could live without and what you could add more of. If there's something on the "bad" list that you don't think you can live without, then try to find a way to make a healthier alternative. I found a great "milkshake" recipe and it's totally good for me. If you need some help in this, check out my website and I will send you a link for a free cookbook.

Lastly, don't be intimidated by the whole "raw" thing. If you aren't sure you can always start with buying prepackaged organic salad, then add more items later.

I know organics are a bit more expensive, but if you start with items that have soft skin, ie, peaches, or are leafy, this is a good start. You will be surprised at how much your budget will change when you stop buying processed foods.

I don't buy meat, so my food budget is now spent in the produce department. All of this may take you awhile. I have just now started buying organic oats, honey and peanut butter to make energy bars. It's just like any project, it may take a bit more when you first get started, but in the long run, you will definitely feel better.

Here's a partial list of foods to try.

Good Fats-

Nuts   Coconut Oil   Olive Oil   Avocados   Salmon
Dark Chocolate!!!!

Proteins

Beans   Fish   Organic Chicken   Nuts

Some vegetables like Kale have protein.

Better Grains- Breads and Pasta

Quinoa   Brown rice   Spelt   Millet

Fresh Organic Fruits and Vegetables

Berries   Bananas   Sweet Potatoes   Leafy Greens

Apples   Peaches   Carrots… well you get the picture. This list goes on and on.

Try to avoid processed foods. Oh and foods with gluten.

Remember to be kind to yourself. This is the new you. As I said earlier, I love to cook. Now I cut a salad or make a juice lovingly, not just for someone else, but for me. Because, doggone it, I'm worth it.

In Conclusion…And Furthermore

"I didn't really say everything I said"-

Yogi Berra

I hate to admit it, but this is my favorite part of a long speech. I have a hard time sitting still and focusing on anything for very long. I will try to make this short and sweet. (No pun intended)

Let me re-cap…. First thing you have to do is make up your mind. Nothing is ever going to change until you change your mind.

Next point, -the reason we are fat and staying that way is because we are in a constant state of abundance. We no longer have to worry about storing up enough fat to sustain us through the famine.

We have to become our own health and food advocate. Not everyone is lucky enough to live with a food Nazi.

Processed foods contain things that can be hazardous to our health. Not too scare anyone or anything, but we have to deal with enough harmful things in the environment as it is. Why would you put extra chemicals and things that contribute to your waistline in your body?

Food addictions are real, learn your own triggers and avoid those as much as possible.

Stop trying to diet. Also, there is no "magic pill". Diet gurus want you to buy their diet or pay for herbs and pills that will fix you.

Instead change the way you think, eat and live. Don't think in terms of denial, think, "I CHOOSE to eat differently." Take back the control of your health.

I recommend reading up on whole grains, GMOs and processed foods for yourself. Make lists of better alternatives and make choices based on what **YOU** find out.

And last but not least, love yourself and your body. Pay attention to what's going on. No one else can know as much about you, as you do.

So…. the #1 little secret? Diets don't work, you have to take control of what you are eating and be your own food and nutrition advocate.

Sources

Hank Cardell-*Stuffed*-Harper Collins 2009

Dr. Michael Roizen and Dr. Mehmet Oz. -*You the Owner's Manual* – Harper Collins 2005.

Documentary- *Hungry for Change*

Documentary-*Food Inc.*

Documentary- *King Corn*

Documentary – *Killer at Large*

http://www.whydontyoutrythis.com/2013/07/new-mri-research-reveals-cancer-cells-thrive-on-processed-sugar.html

http://www.drlwilson.com/articles/butter.htm

http://en.wikipedia.org/wiki/Pink_slime

http://recipes.howstuffworks.com/pinkslime-ammonia-ground-beef.htm

http://www.mercola.com/article/aspartame/symptoms.htm

http://abcnews.go.com/Health/diet-coke-ad-defends-artificial-sweeteners/story?id=19958794

http://www.news-medical.net/news/20120521/Salt-intake-why-is-it-bad-for-you.aspx

About the Author-

Vickie Knob is a mother and grandmother who lives on the Western Slope of Colorado with her husband, three dogs and a very demanding cat. Her first indie published book (the first in the Bathroom Library Series) "The #1 Little Secret to Getting Fit That Trainers Don't Want you to Know" is also available at amazon.com and on kindle.

Sign up for a free e-cookbook or get more information on her website at www.vlknobauthor.com

Please leave a review at Amazon.com thanks so much!